# All you need to know....

# about Tinnitus

Garth Howell

# CONTENTS

The writer      Pg 1

1 What is Tinnitus      Pg ii

2 The causes of Tinnitus      Pg iv

3 The diagnosis of Tinnitus      Pg ix

4 Hearing tests      Pg xi

5 The sounds of Tinnitus      Pg xv

6 Treating Tinnitus      Pg xvii

7 Research      Pg xxv

8 Sleeping with Tinnitus      Pg xxvi

9 Menieres disease      Pg xxiv

10 Summary      Pg xxxi

## THE WRITER

The writer is not a medical practitoner but is an experienced researcher and writer. He has himself suffered from tinnitus at periods of his life although his condition was not too serious. In writing this book the writer sought various opinions from sufferers of this condition.

The intention of this book is not to give medical advice but to help sufferers understand tinnitus and demonstrate that help is available to alleviate the symptoms of the condition.

Thank you for purchasing the book I do hope that that the information contained in it is of help to you.

# All you need to know...about Tinnitus

## What is Tinnitus

Tinnitus is an upleasant condition and is the medical term used to describe the sensation or perception of noise in the sufferers ear, ears or inside the head. The noise is perceived from inside rather than being from an external source. The most simple definition may be any sound that the listener hears that is not in their external environment. The word tinnitus comes from the latin word "tinnire" which means to ring.

Sufferers of tinnitus do not all hear the same type of sound. Many people will describe tinnitus as a ringing sound but some of the other sounds that can be heard are ringing, Humming, whistling, music or buzzing.

The noise associated with tinnitus is sometimes heard with a beat which is in time with the sufferets heartbeat or pulse. This has been called pulsatile tinnitus.

The percieved noises can be worse at different

times, particularly when you are quiet and perhaps you are trying to sleep. It can also be worse if you are fatigued in any way.. The reason for this is because there is less noise around you to cause distraction.

Be aware that tinnitus is a symptom, not a condition and the sounds are almost always only heard by the sufferer. There are a few rare cases when others too have been able to hear it.

There is also a complaint known as temporary tinnitus which may be caused by having a cold, exposure to noise for a prolonged period, or a blow to the head.

# The causes of timmitus

There are several causes of tinnitus but the main one is damage to the inner ear.

When you hear the sounds pass through the external ear canal into the middle ear which it passes through and into the middle ear. The middle ear contains the cochlea and the auditory nerve. The cochlea is a coiled tube in the form of a spiral in which are a large number of very sensitive hair cellswhich are disturbed when the sound disturbes them. The sound are transmitted to the brain via the auditory nerve. If there is any dmage to cochlea or part of it the signal will no longer be sent to the brain as it should. The causes the brain to work harder to find signals from those parts of the cochlea which are still functioning. The brain "over represents these signals and in turn causes the sound known as tinnitus.

The cochlea in fact acts as the "microphone" in us picking up sounds. The necessary adjustments made when we need to react to different sounds are made automatically by nerve signals sent by the part of the brain that handles sound processing.

This makes us very adaptable in picking up the softest of sounds like twig snapping when someone steps on it to being able to pick up one voice out of many in a crowd. This may well be one of the reasons that we get tinnitus.

Tinnitus occurs when the brain realises it is not receiving the full signal it is used to from the cochlear. This in turn sends a signal back down trying to encourage the hair cells that are functioning properly to work harder.

As people get older there can be natural hearing loss as the hair cells in the cochlea either die off or become damaged and this in turn causes the tinnitus to occur. As they can't becaiuse they are damaged the brain tries to get the hair cells to work even harder. This signal back to the hair cells is like a reverse current on a microphone and just cuases them to vibrate thus causing this sound known as tinnitus

There are other causes of tinnitus and even after careful examination by a specialist they can prove difficult to idnetify. However as well as the natural hearing loss there are other possible causes of tinnitus.

A build up of ear wax

An infection of the middle ear known as otis media.

Glue ear

Osteosclerosis. This is inherited and is where there has been abnormal bone growth in the middle ear causing hearing loss.

Menieres disease where the labrynth, part of the inner ear is infected. This can cause problems with balance.

Anaemia. Here the number of red blood cells are reduced thus causing the blood to become thinner and thus circulate more quickly. If it circulates too rapidly it can cause a sound.

Pagets disease which is where there is a disruption to the normal cycle of renewal and repair to the bones in the ear.

Perforation of the eardrum.

Rarer causes of tinnitus can be caused by a blow to the head or some other head injury.

Being exposed to a very loud noise or bang such as an explosion.

Having an adverse reaction to certain medecins such as aspirin, various antibiotics, diuretics or quinine

Solvent or alcohol abuse

Overactive thyroid (hyperthyroidism)

Hypertension (high blood presure)

Acoustic neuroma. This is a non cancerous growth affecting the hearing nerve in the inner ear known as an acoustic neuroma. This is a rare condition.

If you suffer from tinnitus stress can sometimes make it worse but it is not a cause of the condition.

One often thinks that a tinnitus sufferer only hears one sound but it is quite likely that they can hear different sounds, possible in different ears as well, and it is this unpredicatabbility that can make tinnitus such an unpleasant condition which can be very stressful. The stress can make the tinnitus worse and this can place the sufferer in a vicious circle of stress, anxiety tinnitus.

# The diagnosis of tinnitus

If you have any problems with your hearing like buzzing or ringing sounds then it is advisable to see your medical practitioner as soon as possible. Initially they will ask you about the sounds you are hearing and make an examination of you ears.

It is very likely that you will be referred to a specialist and there are various different place where he could send you. These are

The ear nose and throat unit

An audiological medicine department

The audiology unit

For hearing therapy

The problem is that there could be several causes of your tinnitus. The cause could be simple such as ear wax or possible hingh blood pressure which can normally be treated. It is most important to try to find the cause.

You could be referred to an otolaryngologist who

is a specialist dealing with problems of the ears and the larynx. If you are, a number of tests will be carried to to try to identify the cause and he will also look at your medical history for any clues.

The type of tests that are likely to be carried out are, hearing and balance tests, blood tests and x-rays. CT or MRI scans may also be used to help in the diagnosis as they can help look deep into the ear, auditory nerve and brain.

# Hearing Tests

When seeking advice about your ears your medical practitioner will initially ask you a series of questions:-

**Symptoms**

Is there any pain?

Have you tinnitus in one or both ears?

Are you suffering from any vertigo?

Is there any hearing loss?

Are there any previous medical problems?

It is then highly probable that he will look inside your ear using an auriscope, also known as an otiscope.

The practioner will be looking for:-

Ear wax which could be blocking the ear.

Is there any fluid coming out of the ear?

A bulging eardrum which indicates that there could be infected fluid in the middle ear

A retracted ear drum which indiates uninfected fluid in the middle ear (glue ear)

A perforated ear drum- there is a hole in the eardrum which could could be accompanied by infection.

If you are referred to a specialist they are likely to carry out furthe tests

## Pure tone audiometry

Pure tone audiometry (PTA) tests the Hearing in both ears and ustilises a machine known as an audiometer. This produces a range of sounds at differing frequencies and volumes. It is usual to listen through headphones and respond by pressing a button.

## Speech perception test

This tests the persons ability to hear words without any visual assistance. The words spoken may be played through headphones or a loudspeaker or just spoken by the tester.

The speech test me also be carried out in the presence of some background noise, the noise and type of which is controlled.

## The whispered voice test

The test is very simple and involves your medical practitioner whispering words at differing volumes usually one ear at a time with the other ear blocked. The person being tested will be asked to repeat the words as they hear them.

## The tuning fork test

A tuning fork will be tapped to produce a sound at a fixed pitch. To carry out this test the tester will place a vibratiing tuning ork at each side of the head alongside the ear and also against the mastoid bone which is the bone located just behind the ear. This will help identify the type of any hearing loss.

The test is known as the Rinne test.

The tuning fork may also be placed on the cebtre of the forehead or on the centre of the nose. This test which also helps in identifying the type of hearing loss is known as the Weber test.

## Bone conduction test

This is very much a routine test and is a more sophisticated version of the tuning fork test. Its object is to test how well sounds are heard when transmitted through the bone.

It is carried out using a vibrating probe which held against the mastoid bone.

This test, used in conjunction with pure tone auidometry tests where any hearing problem may lie and whether hearing loss is caused by a problem with the inner or outer ear, or perhaps both.

# The sounds of tinnitus

People suffering with tinnitus experience noise in either one or both ears and the noise heard can take many forms
The type of noise can vary between individuals as can the volume.

## The pitch
The pitch of tinnitus can be a high frquency sound, a whistling, ringing or hissing.
The pitch can be of a low frequency either rumbling, buzzing or roaring
The pitch can also vary.

## The volume
The volume of tinnitus can be very loud or it can be quiet and it can also be variable.
People ability to tolerate these noises varies between suffers. Some have quite a high threshold to noise whereas others are driven to distraction by just a small amount of noise.

## Does tinnitus last long?

The sounds of tinnitus can be very short and just last for a few seconds or they can last for your lifetime. It depends on the individual. Tinnitus may therefore be a permanent condition and you may need to adjust your life accordingly. It may however disappear.

Often however people with permanent tinnitus find that the sounds disappear over time and will only be noticed if you listen for it.

If you are hearing voices then it is not tinnitus, and you should seek medical help

# Treating tinnitus

## Deal with any underlying health problem

If your tinnitus is caused some underlying health problem such as high blood pressure or earwax then solving that particular problem should help the tinnitus.

In most cases however there is no cure and treatment involves helping the sufferer to manage the condition of a daily basis. If you go to a hearing clinic they should work with you to help you to devise an appropriate strategy for management.

### Deal with hearing loss

If you have a hearing problem it is important that it is addressed as it will mean that the parts of the brain occuoied with hearing do not have to work so hard. This in turn should help the tinnitus.

In addition if you can now hear sounds better this should override the tinnitus thus reducing the problem.

## Using sound as therapy

It is usual to not tinnitus more when you are in a quiet environment. Sound therapy involves filling that quiet with neutral sound to act as a distraction.

One way to do this is to have the radio or television on quietly playing in the background.

You could however use a sound generator which produces a soft natural sound such as a babbling brook or waves lapping onto the shore. This could be useful if you have trouble sleeping. You have it switched on by your bed as this could distract you away from the tinnitus as you try to sleep. Some have timers built in so that it will switch off after a set period.

Some hearing aids actually have inbuilt

sound generators to aid the masking of tinnitus.

## Cognitive behavioural therapy

Cognitive behavioural therapy (CBT) tries to help you change the way you act and think to provide assistance in solving problems. It tackles any problem in two main ways.

1. To think and talk about yourself, other people, and the world in general

2. How your actions affect what you think, and how you feel.

Therefore by talking about your tinnitus you can benefit altering the way you think about it, and in in turn change the way you deal with it. It aims to dramatically improve your state of mind.

CBT normally will involve a number of sessions either weekly or fortnightly over a period of time usually varying from 6 weeks to 6 months. Individuals will have differing needs for their treatment.

CBT won't make the tinnitus disappear but it should help the sufferer to be able to live with the condition more easily.

**Prevent further damage caused by noise**

It is important to try to avoid doing any further damage to the hair cells in the cochlear. Keep clear of excessive noise. Remember petrol machines like strimmers and hedge cutters can produce sounds of 85 decibels and pneumatic drills much more. Try to avoid these types of sounds, even for short periods and if you are exposed to the sounds of such machinery then use ear protectors.

**Tinnitus Counselling**

Counselling can be of great help to sufferers

of tinnitus. Just being able to talk to someone about the way you feel can give the sufferer reassurance. There are several types of counselling available and these are:-

## Medical couselling

This is where you speak to a medical specialist who really has an understanding of how the condition can affect the sufferer. The mdical counsellor can help by alleviating any fears, helping the sufferer to understand what is happening, showing you that there are other sufferes and also helping you to live with it. It is a part of the treatment known as Tinnituus retraining therapy.

## Private counselling

Private counselling involves speaking to a counsellor who operates privately or through a counselling agency. It can be very helpful if you have stressful problems with your life which may be making your tinnitus worse. Talking through your problems can be very helpful and can help your tinnitus.

It is important to select your counsellor carefully as their qualifications and experience can vary greatly. If you are trying to find a counsellor it is advisable to chack with a one of the professional bodies for counsellors.

## Lay counselling

The lay counsellor is not formally qualified but should have experience and received some training. Their experience of life can be very useful and the lay counsellor could be a member of a local support group and may even be a sufferer themselves.

## Group counselling

Your medical adviser my recommend that you participate in a group session. Here, several itnnitus sufferers meet together and talk through their problems and difficulties. The aim is help the participants learn how to handle their problem by talking it through with others who are having to meet similar challenges.

## Tinnitus retraining therapy (TRT)

This treatment for tinnitus involves the utilisation of counselling and some sound therapy to aid sufferers to cope better and to cease the negative reaction to the sound and to reduce the perception of it.

TRT involves retraining the brain so that it filters or tunes out the sound of the Tinnitus so that the suffer is less aware of it. This is known as habituation.

It is not usually used in its full form as it is a complex technique, but is used in a less structured way. This treatment should only be given by a suitably trained professional.

## Self help

Some tinnitus sufferers are able to control their condition by using a few simple self help techniques.

These could be:-

1. Using relaxation techniques. These can help you to avoid stress and help you to relax. Such activities could involve yoga, deep breathing or walking.
2. Listening to music. Relaxing music not only can relax you but also mask the effects of the tinnitus
3. You may find belonging to a local suppoert group is helpful. There may well be one in your locality and it could be worthwhile you seeking it out and talking with people who have the same problem as you do.

**Medication**

There is no specific tinnitus medication but you may be treated for any anxiety or depression as a result of it with antidepressants or tranqilisers. This could be in conjuntion with couselling or other types of treatment.

## Research

At the time of wrting this book research is being carried out to produce a drug which will help to regulate the damaged cells which cause the tinnitus. The drug is being developed to stop the erratic firing of the cells and return them to their normal resting state. The research is still in its early stage and the treatment could still be some years away.

# Sleeping with Tinnitus

We have already touched on this subject of the difficulty tinnitus sufferers have in getting to sleep. For tinnitus sufferers it can be a bit like trying to sleep on a motorway verge, or in a large shopping mall when they are busy. It is really difficult and it most certainly isn't fun.

So if it is a major problem just how do you get to sleep. It is most important that you get sleep as sleep starvation may make your tinnitus appear worse because you are concentrating on it and of course sleep deprivation can make you ill.

There are however steps that you can take which should help ensure that you get a good nights sleep.

Firstly ensure that you are tired. Make sure that you really need to sleep when you take to your bed.

Avoid watching television just before you retire for the night. The last thing you need is your head filled with information and your brain buzzing with activity before you sleep.

Don't raise your adrenalin levels by taking exercise before you go to bed. You don't want you heart racing and high energy levels when you are trying to sleep.

Don't eat after 8p.m. To ensure your digestive system is not working overtime avoid taking in products that can have an adverse reaction on your tinnitus like alcohol and caffeine.

It may help to learn to meditate and practice this just before going to bed. Try deep breathing. It will help you to relax.

Work on relaxation techniques and use them when lying in bed.

Ensure that you are lying in a quiet dark well ventilated room. If you have any noise ensure it is natural noise like lapping waves or rustling trees.

If all else fails perhaps try sex!!!!

# Menieres disease

Menieres disease is a rare disorder affeting the inner ear. It can cause a feeling of pressure in the inner ear along with tinnitus, hearing loss and possibly loss of balance.

The symptoms which can appear without warning can last for several hours and the symptoms may take 2 or 4 days to completely go away. The symptoms differ widely between individuals .

There is known known cause of Menieres disease but it is believed to be caused by a problem with pressure in the inner ear.

The condition goes through different stages and in its early stage sufferer can endure 6-11 attacks per year but this reduces and the symptoms should improve and disappear after about 2-8 years. Some peopale however may be left with permanent hearing loss in one or both ears and this may or not be accompanied by tinnitus.

There is no single cure of Menieres disease and wide variety of treatments may be used such as medication to both treat and prevent attacks, treatment for anxiety and physiotherapy to help balance. Treatment for tinnitus may also be given as well as dietary advice. Salt does seem to have an effect on Menieres disease and the sufferer may be advised to go on a low salt diet.

# Summary

To sum up, tinnitus is quite a common complaint and causes much stress and anxiety to the sufferer.

It is well worthwhile seeking advice from your medical practitioner who even if they are not able to advise can act by directing you to an ear nose and throat specialist or some other expert who will be able to help.

It is also worthwhile to seek advice because the tinnitus may well be a symptom of some other underlying but as yet undiagnosed condition which if diagnosed and treated will cause the tinnitus to disappear as well.
If however this is not the case then it is worth a specialist trying to find the cause of your tinnitus to see if he can help.

It is possible that there will be no cure for your tinnitus but in almost all cases help can be given that will help the stress and ansiety and help the sufferer to be less aware of the condition.

If you are a tinnitus sufferer then please seek help, I am sure that it will be worth the effort.